A PAEDIATRIC CATECHISM

A PAEDIATRIC CATECHISM

Graham Clayden
MD, FRCP

Honorary Consultant Paediatrician,
St Thomas's Hospital, London

HODDER AND STOUGHTON
LONDON   SYDNEY   AUCKLAND   TORONTO

Typeset by Rowland Phototypesetting Ltd,
Bury St Edmunds, Suffolk

Printed in Great Britain for Hodder and Stoughton Educational,
a division of Hodder and Stoughton Ltd,
Mill Road, Dunton Green, Sevenoaks, Kent TN13 2YD
by Richard Clay Ltd, Bungay, Suffolk

CONTENTS

INTRODUCTION

OVERALL AIMS

The purpose of this book is to provide paediatric students with a guide to history taking and physical examination which will help them during training and in preparing for their examinations. It focuses on helping students to associate key symptoms and signs with the diagnosis of common problems in childhood. There is deliberate emphasis on how childrens' problems differ from those of adults. Stress is laid on the importance of empathy and communication skills when meeting children with their parents.

It is aimed to provide some support for students who often feel that their uncertainty of what to ask or what to do when clerking patients interferes with their rapport and confidence.

A systematic path is taken through details of the history taking and physical examination with advice on organizing your findings. Many examiners in undergraduate and postgraduate clinical examinations complain bitterly about the disorganization of the candidates' technique. It is hoped that this small book will provide a formal structure which will help you disabuse these critics and therefore lead you to success in these clinical examinations.

It is also hoped that by having a fluent style, many vital routines will become second nature and help the practising doctor to avoid missing essential elements of the consultation and examination during periods in professional life when time is the major constraint.

HOW TO USE THIS BOOK OR HOW TO BENEFIT MOST FROM CLERKING YOUR CHILD PATIENTS

When you are reading this book try to imagine yourself at the bedside of the child, with his or her parents. Rehearse in your mind how you would incorporate what you are reading into the way you respond to the clinical situation. In this way you will be able to approach your child patients with more confidence and avoid missing useful clinical experience by being reticent for the first few weeks of your paediatric clinical attachment.

It is hoped that this book will encourage you to develop an active learning style. If you involve yourself in the real life situation which your patient and the family are going through, it will provide you with a personal insight and broaden your experience. As it is a vivid experience it will act as a valuable centre of association for a number of facts related to the disease which might be difficult to memorize on their own. So getting to know your patient is not only good practice for your future career but it can act as a reference point for learning and remembering those facts which may be tested in your final examinations.

THE HISTORY

When you are taking the history you must find the balance between conversation and interrogation. Your social introduction is important and may be considered under these headings:

1 WELCOME
2 REQUEST
3 POSITIONING AND POSTURE
4 EYE CONTACT
5 SHARING ATTENTION—CHILD/PARENTS
6 CHAT VERSUS INFORMATION ACQUISITION
7 INTERRUPTION
8 CLOSING AND LEAVING

WELCOME

Introduce yourself and explain why you are there. Ascertain who you are talking to; a friendly method is to check you know your patient's first name and his relationship with any adult present. This information can be obtained from the nurses, whose permission you must seek before approaching the child for the first time. This is not only courtesy but may help you to avoid embarrassing situations. For example, saying 'Hello, Jimmy and hello, you must be Jimmy's granny' and then getting a stony look and the reply, 'I'm Jamie and this is my mother.'

REQUEST

Your request to ask a few questions and perform a basic examination will rarely be denied but it is essential you do ask and not assume a divine right to do so.

POSITIONING AND POSTURE

Try to avoid towering over children or putting either a desk or a bed between you and them. This will reduce the formality and also allow you and them to speak more quietly, thus reducing the risk of eavesdroppers. It is important to appreciate confidentiality in this way as well as avoiding talking about your patients in public areas or with non medical colleagues.

EYE CONTACT

Even if you feel shy try to overcome the tendency to bury your head in your notes. Eye contact will reassure your patient and allow you to detect early signs that you are on a topic which is upsetting or embarrassing.

SHARING ATTENTION

The child is your patient and depending on his or her maturity and interest, you should address your questions and eye contact towards him. The parent will have details which may not be recalled by the child. It is relatively easy to speak with both simultaneously provided you are aware of the need to involve the child even if he is relatively silent. A request for a clarification or more details of a particular symptom is easier for a child to answer than a very open-ended question.

CHAT VERSUS INFORMATION ACQUISITION

When you are getting started a general question to the child and parent such as 'What brought you here?' will usually initiate the discussion on the present complaint. If the child says 'an ambulance' you will have to judge whether or not he is joking and continue appropriately. It will depend on the nature of the illness and the time you have available whether the conversation is free flowing or structured. A reasonable rule of thumb is that the more surgical the more structured.

INTERRUPTION

Interrupting is sometimes necessary to steer the discussion away from what you find is an irrelevant area. However, caution is required to avoid offence and you must also be sure that you do not miss an area of the history that they may be moving towards. Interruption to clarify a point is usually acceptable provided it does not indicate that you think they are expressing themselves badly.

CLOSING AND LEAVING

This again requires the same tact as closing any conversation. Thanking the child and family and making plans to continue at another time together with a reason why you are having to leave is helpful. In an exam it is worth checking with the child or parent a brief summary of the history as any misunderstanding can then be corrected. It is also valuable practice for the initial contact with the examiner. For example, 'Jamie has a five year history of recurrent wheezing and was admitted with an acute attack two days ago in spite of regular medication at home'.

THE HISTORY—PRESENTING SYMPTOMS

The range of presenting symptoms is obviously enormous and beyond the scope of this small book. However, in paediatrics the incidence differs from that of general medicine. For example, vomiting is very common but haematemesis much less so; failure to thrive, developmental delay, precocious or delayed puberty, parental neglect or child abuse are classic problems of childhood. The age of the child is of vital importance in diagnosis as disease has characteristic age related incidence.

DEFINING THE PRESENTING SYMPTOM

The following features of the presenting symptom should be obtained during the history taking:

Onset
sudden
gradual
following a more minor symptom, e.g. a febrile convulsion after mild malaise

Duration
An estimate of time elapsed from onset to presentation. This may be difficult for patient or parent to recall but if they can relate it to a more definite event it may help

Previous attacks

Treatment already given for this complaint

Details
The easiest symptom to define in detail is probably pain where the following are usually reasonably accurately describable, except in very young children:

1 **Anatomical site:** most children will point to the site
2 **Radiation:** most will respond to the question 'Where does it go?'
3 **Character:** 'Aching, burning, colicky, stabbing?'

4 **Relieved by/aggravated by:** 'Does anything make it
better/worse?' e.g.:
drinking or eating
defaecation
micturition
changing posture
sleeping
rubbing

5 **Associated symptoms,** e.g.:
nausea
jaundice
diarrhoea
altered consciousness
vomiting
urinary frequency
constipation

The following table gives examples of common painful childhood
problems and shows how the symptom grid may help.

Illness	Site of pain	Radiation of pain	Character of pain	Relieved by	Aggravated by	Associated with
Appendicitis	central abdomen	RIF later	severe ache	nil	movement, touching especially PR	nausea vomiting anorexia
Urinary tract infection	loin	perineum	often colicky	moving	passing urine usually	frequency dysuria rigors
Pneumonia (pleurisy)	chest	abdomen shoulder	stabbing	nil	breathing coughing	tachypnoea cough
Meningitis	head	neck	severe ache	lumbar puncture later	light moving	vomiting altered conscious- ness/fits
Migraine	head abdomen in young	nil	ache	sleep	light moving	vomiting visual- effects
Raised intra- cranial pressure	head	variable	severe ache variable	upright posture	sleep	morning- vomiting vision affected
Osteo- myelitis	local	local	exquisite pain	nil	moving touching	malaise fever
Otitis media	ear	variable	severe	occasional swallow	touching	deafness fever

RIF = Right iliac fossa
PR = Per rectum examination

Other painful conditions can also be fitted into such a table and it would be a useful exercise to continue this table yourself for conditions such as sickle cell disease, intussusception, mumps, anal fissure, cellulitis, juvenile arthritis, etc.

So far, we have considered the presenting symptom from its onset, duration and details which included looking closely at pain. Certain other symptoms will lead to a cascade of associated questions as in the case of pain. Here are some other examples:

1 **Vomiting:**
age of onset
projectile
bile stained
abdominal distension
pain
headache

2 **Convulsions:**
length of fit
generalized or localized
fever preceding onset
post ictal behaviour

3 **Itch:**
other atopic features
contact? scabies
       chickenpox
generalized (eczema)/local (pruritis ani)

4 **Fever with rash:**
time relationship between onset of fever and rash
contact history and timing (compare with incubation period)
immunization status

A useful mnemonic for the relationship between the onset of the fever and the appearance of the rash is: 'Really Sick People Must Take No Exercise'.

Interval in days from onset of fever to rash:	1	2	3	4	5	6	7
Initial letter:	R	S	P	M	T	N	E
Infection:	Rubella	Scarlet Fever	Pox (Small Pox)	Measles	Typhus	None for day 6	Enteric fevers

The other classical association between fever and rash is **roseola infantum**, a viral infection where the rash appears within a day of the fever subsiding. It is a very common illness in children under 2 years of age.

Working out the relationship between symptoms is always useful. Associations between the major symptoms presenting in childhood are particularly valuable, and we will be considering them in the section on the Systematic Enquiry (see p. 10). However, if fever and rash had been the presenting symptoms, these questions should be asked at the same time as defining the present complaint.

THE HISTORY—SYSTEMATIC ENQUIRY

It is useful for the sake of continuity to follow on from the history of the present complaint with a systematic enquiry starting with the most relevant system of the body. This helps with logical thought and avoids confusing the child and parents.

The systematic enquiry in paediatrics has a different emphasis from that in general medicine. More details are required in relation to nutrition, developmental progress, behaviour and sleep patterns. Time and attention should be given to those areas where the child or parent shows particular concern. You will have more time available to take a full history than the Senior House Officer or Registrar have, so it is likely that you will receive information and evidence of family anxiety which may have been hidden from or missed by the others. Your role in the team will be confirmed when you pass this information on so that reassurance or further investigation can be set in motion. It is important that you do not try to explain the intricacies of the child's problem even if you have a clear view of it, because there may be other factors which you may not have been aware of. A discussion with the doctors looking after the child will benefit all sides.

QUESTIONS RELATED TO GENERAL HEALTH
Alertness
Activity
Tendency to recurrent nonspecific illness
Ability to recovery from minor illnesses

QUESTIONS RELATED TO PHYSICAL DEVELOPMENT AND NUTRITION
Weight gain (evidence from Child Health Clinic cards or booklets)
Appetite
Food and milk intake (depending on age)
Food fads
Eating behaviour

GASTRO-INTESTINAL SYSTEM

1 **Vomiting**

Subsidiary questions:

more than possetting	—normal?
bile	—obstructed?
blood	—oesophagitis?
long delay since meal	—pyloric stenosis?
pain association	—intussusception?
pleasure association	—rumination
particular food	—intolerance?
abdominal distension	—Hirschsprungs?
associated steatorrhoea	—coeliac?
associated tenderness	—appendicitis?
associated headache	—migraine?
	—raised intracranal pressure?

Feeding problems are more common than any of the suggested disorders and may be associated with maternal postnatal depression.

2 **Diarrhoea**

This term is often used loosely with stools ranging from so liquid they soak through a nappy to stools softer than normal. It is important to ask how liquid they are.

Subsidiary questions:

acute and vomiting	—gastroenteritis?
food related	—intolerance?
failure to thrive	—coeliac/cystic fibrosis?

3 **Constipation**

Again a term used variably usually meaning delay and difficulty in passing a stool. Many use the term to indicate a hard stool.

Subsidiary questions:

acute	
chronic with blood PR	—anal fissure?
overflow soiling	—megacolon?
neonatal onset	—anal stenosis/Hirschsprungs?

4 **Jaundice**

The age of the child is important. Neonatal jaundice is considered in the past medical history (see p. 15). Persistent jaundice with failure to thrive is suspicious of liver disease (biliary atresia or neonatal hepatitis).

Jaundice with anorexia and vomiting is suggestive of infective hepatitis especially if there has been foreign travel or other contact.

RESPIRATORY SYSTEM

1 **Cough**
Subsidiary questions:
night mainly
exercise related
sputum
2 **Wheeze**
Subsidiary questions:
night mainly
exercise related
allergen contact
3 **Croup/stridor**

EAR, NOSE AND THROAT

1 **Ear infections** (recurrent earache)
2 **Deafness** (may be inferred from speech delay)
3 **Nocturnal snoring**
4 **Sore throats**
5 **Epistaxes**

CARDIOVASCULAR SYSTEM

1 **Activity**
   Subsidiary questions:
   exercise tolerance
2 **Colour changes**
   Subsidiary questions:
   blue attacks
   pallor
3 **Breathlessness**
4 **Recurrent chest infections**
5 Has a **heart murmur** been heard at a routine examination?

GENITO-URINARY SYSTEM

1 **Urinary infections**
   Subsidiary questions:
   proven bacteriological
   recurrent

2 **Frequency**
3 **Urgency**
4 **Urinary incontinence**
   Subsidiary questions:
   daytime
   stress/giggle related
   nocturnal enuresis

SKIN

1 **Eczema**
2 **Nappy rash**
3 **Other rashes**
   Subsidiary questions:
   petechial
   blisters
4 **Hair problems**
   Subsidiary questions:
   total hair loss
   child eating hair
   infestations

LOCOMOTOR SYSTEM

1 **Joint pain**
2 **Joint swelling/redness**
3 **Joint stiffness**
4 **Limping**
5 **Limb pains**

CENTRAL NERVOUS SYSTEM

1 **Convulsions** If the child has attacks which are described as convulsions, seizures or fits, it is valuable to analyse the parents' description of the attack under the following headings:

Aura or warning state
Length of loss of consciousness
Falling down
Grand mal progression (aura-tonic-clonic-post ictal)
Localized or generalized
Post ictal state

This table will show how these features help to discriminate the common 'attacks' of childhood.

'Attack' type	Warning of onset	Duration of fit	Falls down?	Progression of movement	Local/ generalized	State after fit
Grand mal epilepsy	aura	long	yes	classical	often unilateral	confused or sleeping
Febrile convulsion	fever	brief usually	yes	incomplete	generalized	alert but hot
Breath-holding	angry screaming	unconscious briefly		rare	limp	normal
Faint	dizzy pallor	brief no fit	yes	nil	limp	normal
Petit mal	nil	seconds only	no	eyes stare	nil	normal

Each of the attacks listed above are very distressing to the parents, especially the one who witnesses it first; they may even feel the child has actually died. It will be valuable for you to enquire about how they felt when it happened. This will be both instructive for you and it will reinforce the communication between you and the parent.

2 **Headaches**
   Subsidiary questions:
   time of day—morning in raised ICP
   visual effects—migraine
   upper respiratory infections—sinus
   upset or tense—tension headaches

3 **Vision**

4 **Balance and coordination**

5 **Muscles**
   Subsidiary questions:
   pain/weakness—muscular dystrophy
   unilateral—hemiplegia
   motor skills—sitting
              —crawling
              —walking

PAST MEDICAL HISTORY

Details of past illnesses and operations should be recorded as in general medicine. However, with children, the maternal obstetric history and the neonatal history are very important.

Did mother have an infectious disease in early pregnancy?
   ?rubella ?toxoplasmosis ?cytomegalo virus ?AIDS
Has she an illness which may have affected the foetus?
   ?diabetes ?thyrotoxicosis ?hypertension
Had she been on medication or drugs?
   ?anticonvulsants ?narcotics ?excess alcohol ?smoking

   Tact is especially required in asking these questions as parents often feel responsible for their child's illness even if this is not justified medically.

Was there birth asphyxia/ need for resuscitation?
Was the baby born before term?
Was the baby an appropriate weight for the gestational age?
Were there any of the common neonatal problems and with what severity?
   ?respiratory distress ?jaundice ?infection ?convulsions

Other questions should also be asked at this point:

Early feeding
   ?breast ?how long ?age weaned to solids
Sleeping patterns
Immunization history
Serious illnesses, hospital admissions and operation

   Sometimes development is included in the Past Medical History and sometimes it is given as a separate section of the history.

DEVELOPMENTAL HISTORY

Development can be considered in four main domains:

Gross motor
Head control
Sitting unsupported
Crawling
Walking around furniture (cruising)
Walking unaided
Walking backwards
Hopping

Hand eye coordination
Reaches out for objects
How the baby picks up objects
How many bricks can be built up

Language
Cooing
Babbling
Mimicking words
Using words
Linking words in phrases then sentences

Social
Neonatal eye regard
Smiling
Feeding himself
Helping with tasks like dressing
Playing in parallel with other children
Playing with other children

FAMILY HISTORY

Here is an opportunity to discover useful information for establishing a diagnosis as well as getting to know the child's position within the structure of the family. Tact is required since many families have complicated relationships, some of which may be unknown to the child. It is valuable to draw a chart of the family, using the standard symbols and generation divisions. Here are some examples of how a detailed knowledge of the family tree helps in recognizing Mendelian inherited disorders:

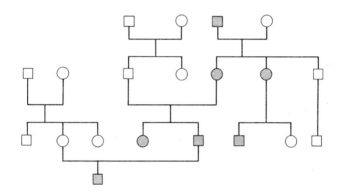

Note the affected member(s) in each generation with no sex discrimination—characteristic of autosomal dominant inheritance as seen in:

Achondroplasia
Neurofibromatosis
Tuberose sclerosis
Dystrophia myotonica
Osteogenesis imperfecta

17

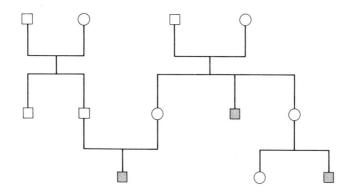

Note here how only the males are affected and some generations spared, with the females passing on the affected X chromosome—typical of X-linked recessive conditions:

Haemophilia
Christmas disease
Duchenne muscular dystrophy
Colour blindness

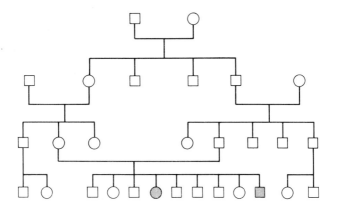

Note how in this pedigree the consanguinous cousin marriage allowed the autosomal recessive gene to become manifest. Disorders of this type include:

Cystic fibrosis
Congenital adrenal hyperplasia
Phenylketonuria
Albinism
Tay-Sac's disease
Sickle cell anaemia

The chances of individuals carrying a single gene vary between ethnic groups, for example in Caucasians the carrier rate for cystic fibrosis is approximately 1 in 25. Thus, for a common recessive trait consanguinity is less likely.

Other familial traits occur but not following single gene genetics, but still knowledge of a positive family history would help clarify the diagnosis e.g. atopy, diabetes mellitus, auto immune disease, febrile convulsions.

Other useful points can be obtained from the family history:

Age and sex of siblings
Heights of parents
Whether both parents are living together
Whether the parents are ill
Whether siblings have any illness which they may fear this child has, or which may distract normal attention from this child.

SOCIAL HISTORY

The social history has a very important significance in the problems of childhood. The child shares the emotional and environmental stresses of the family. The family's capacity to partner the professionals in the management of the problems will depend on a number of variables which may be elicited by an accurate social history. It is very damaging to err in either direction when it comes to deciding how much support the family needs in coping with the medical problems.

Important areas need to be covered with tact and the interviewer must think ahead when questioning in sensitive areas. It is upsetting to the development of rapport when a parent refuses to provide information, for example the details of marital breakdown or the child's parentage, to a student in an open ward setting. The social history is best obtained by a structured interview technique using open-ended questions as prompts. This may be illustrated by the following questions and the information which will probably be volunteered:

1 **Do you have any problems with housing?**
    own/council/private rented
    house/maisonette/flat
    high rise/garden
    isolated/difficult neighbourhood
    damp/damaged/cold
    moving soon/settled
2 **Are you still going out to work?**
    full-time job/part-time job/full-time mother
    child minder/creche/nursery
    relative/nanny looks after child when mother works
    mother's occupation
    enjoys/puts up with/hates
3 **What does the other parent do?**
    unemployed/works away from home/home late/overworks

type of work
financial problems

4 **Has the child adapted to these arrangements?**
relationships with the above

5 **How is he/she getting on at school** (depending on age)?
name of school/nursery etc
ordinary/special help
educational progress
relationship with other children
school refusal
teachers helping with symptoms or treatments

6 **How does he/she get on with any siblings?**
only child/last born etc
jealousy/rivalry/aggression
isolated

7 **What sort of temperament has he/she?**
easily frightened—shy/cries easily—sad/easily
angered—aggressive/boisterous—overactive

8 **How does he/she get on with you and partner?**
tantrums/disobedience
overdependent/independent
disagreement on management

NB The partner who brings up the child may be the spouse but
is often a grandparent and conflicts of management may echo
difficulties in the parent's own childhood.

9 **Has he/she got into trouble at school or with the law?**
trouble in classroom
truanting
trouble with police

10 **Has there been any professional help given about
behaviour?**
health visitor/social worker/GP/paediatrician/child
psychiatrist
ongoing help

11 **Are you a happy family?**
marital problems
financial problems
psychiatric illnesses
drug/alcohol problems

From question 4 onwards this becomes the **behaviour** or **psychological** history of the child. These sections may be considered with the **developmental** history or the CNS section of the **systematic** enquiry. It does however fit quite well into the discussion with the parent and child, starting from fairly neutral subjects such as housing, going on to more sensitive issues such as relationships. It is debatable how much of this should be discussed in the presence of the child. This depends on age but it must be considered that if children are excluded from a discussion they will probably assume that serious or frightening issues are being covered.

COMPLETION OF HISTORY

Closing the discussion on the social/behavioural history must be done with attention to how the child and family are feeling. One way of moving the discussion to more neutral ground is to ask if there are any other points about the symptoms or illness you should know about before going on to the physical examination

THE PHYSICAL EXAMINATION

The physical examination must be adapted to suit the age and sensitivity of the individual child. This may mean that certain examination procedures will have to be taken out of the traditional order. One of the main reasons for having a definite plan in examining a system is to avoid missing whole areas and leaving out essential elements in the examination. In the following pages advice is given on how to follow an ordered procedure. However, frequently the more unpopular examinations such as looking in the ears are best left to the last.

It may be far from ideal to examine a child other than on the examination couch. If, however, he or she is potentially afraid of leaving the parent's lap your examination must be carefully adapted.

If you approach the child from his own level rather than towering above him, he is less likely to be afraid. It is often said that paediatricians share the 'baggy-kneed-suit sign' with priests as a result of years of kneeling to examine toddlers.

Sometimes performing a brief mock examination of a nearby doll or cuddly toy may allay the child's fears. Allowing the child to handle the stethoscope is often reassuring although it may be difficult for you to retrieve it. If you smile and talk to small children as you approach to examine them they are less likely to find you a threat. Unfortunately there is a tendency to overdo this which may amuse the child but destabilize your rapport with the parents. If you appear tense and anxious the child will sense this and react in sympathy. It is always important to wash one's hands prior to examination; it is even more vital when examining babies. Remember to wash in warm water as there is nothing more likely to lead to loss of cooperation than your icy hands touching the warm infant skin.

Although it is important to expose the area to be examined for effective inspection, children and especially adolescents are very easily embarrassed. Care should be taken to screen off the bed or couch and, depending on the culture of the child, the parent may or may not expect to be present. For example, girls from some cultures may be deeply offended by having to undress in the presence of their fathers or brothers. However, if the parent is not with the child a chaperone is essential, so that your examinations are not misunderstood. This is further evidence of the need to check with the nursing staff before starting your examination of children on the wards. It is far better to wait until the parent is present so they can give consent for your examination and moral support to their child.

PRACTICE FOR CLINICAL EXAMS

When you are examining your child patients allocated to you on your paediatric firms, it is wise to use that opportunity as practice for the final clinical exam. Most exams have short case sections where you may be asked to examine a particular system or area of the body. If you have a clearly defined plan for performing the clinical examination of your patient and you practice using it, you will know where to start even with the surge of adrenaline rising. Some medical schools are introducing Objectively Structured Clinical Examinations (OSCE) into the formal assessment of students. This will emphasize the need for a structured approach to examining for physical signs.

The traditional guide to clinical examination is based on the following stages:

Inspection Local, general, observe movements, instrumental
Palpitation Local, lymphatic drainage, pulses, liver, spleen, PR, etc
Percussion Chest, abdominal, skull
Auscultation Heart, lungs, skull, arteries, blood pressure

It is a valuable exercise to construct check lists based on this structure for every area of the body and then use them. The practised fluency in examination this will lead to will not only impress those evaluating you but will help you to avoid missing out vital sections of your examination when you are a harrassed time-starved clinician.

The following chapters will be laid out according to this plan but it must be repeated that for younger children it may be necessary to stray from it to avoid potentially disrupting your patient's cooperation.

THE GENERAL APPEARANCE

Obviously after having taken a history you will be cued to look for particular physical signs. However there may be additional or even incidental findings which are important. In the short case in a clinical exam you may have no history to help you.

These are the questions which you should be attempting to answer when observing the general appearance of the child:

1 **Does the child look ill?**
   Is there:
   paucity of spontaneous movements
   lack of interest in surroundings or events
   pallor
   irritability or excessive crying: in pain?
   difficulty in breathing
2 **Is the child well cared for?**
   Consider:
   state of hygiene
   condition of clothes
   parental attention or concern
   evidence of child abuse—watchful attentiveness
                           —unusual bruising
                           —flinching
                           —over-friendliness/appeasing
                             gestures
3 **Is the child a normal size for his/her age?**
It is essential to know the precise age, height and weight when examining a child. Reference is then made to a height and weight centile chart to plot the child's relative size compared to children at that age. The position of the child's present plot on the graph is useful but the gradient of several serial plots gives even more useful information.

The figure below plots several examples superimposed on a chart. In practice each child should have an individual chart. On most charts in common use the sloping nearly parallel lines are, from top to bottom, the 97th, 90th, 75th, 50th, 25th, 10th, 3rd centiles. Sometimes only the 90th, 50th and 10th are shown. When plotting the points for babies allowance must be made for preterm delivery.

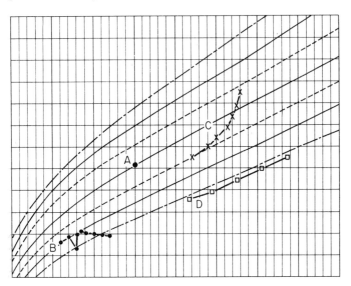

Examples are as follows:
- A An average size child (50th centile)
- B A child initially thriving but now failing to thrive after an acute weight losing episode (as seen with secondary lactose intolerance following gastroenteritis)
- C A child whose weight crosses centile lines upwards (obesity)
- D A small child who is growing parallel to the line (as seen in Turner syndrome)

4 **Does the child look unusual?**

Is there:

unusual facial appearance—Down's syndrome
                             —hypothyroid
                             —hyperthyroid

unusual colour—cyanosis
    —jaundice
unusual pigmentation—tuberose sclerosis
        —neurofibromatosis
        —Addison's disease
unusual posture or movements—cerebral palsy
unusual facial swelling—mumps
        —nephrotic syndrome

5 **Does the child behave unusually?**

Is there:
excessive activity or restlessness
lack of parental control
poor social responsiveness—visual handicap
            — deaf
            —autistic
            —severe retardation
            —depressed

EXAMINATION OF THE FEBRILE CHILD

The examination of a child with a fever is a frequent clinical occurrence. They may have presented with a febrile convulsion or may not have been eating or feeding normally. In practice there is often little time available for a systematic examination and so one looks for major physical signs of the diseases which need urgent attention, e.g. meningitis, septicaemia, acute epiglottitis, peritonitis. However, the inspection/palpation/percussion/auscultation sequence is still valid.

INSPECTION

1 **How ill are they?** (see p. 26)
2 **Meningism:**
   neck stiffness   (all unreliable
   photophobia   in young
   Kernig's sign   children)
3 **Facial swelling:**
   mumps affecting salivary glands plus local facial swelling
4 **Lymphadenopathy:**
   tonsillitis
   infectious mononucleosis (often palatal petechiae)
5 **Redness over bone or joint:**
   osteomyelitis
   septic arthritis
   pseudoparalysis
6 **Tachypnoea:**
   pneumonia
7 **Throat inflammation:**
   tonsillitis
8 **Auroscopy**
   otitis media
9 **Rash**
   see page 8 for relationship between onset of fever and onset of rash

The table below covers some of the useful differences between the infectious disease signs.

Infection	Type of rash	Distribution	Enanthem	Other signs
Measles	macular/ papular	face, spreading down body	Koplic's spots	conjunctivitis cough
Rubella	macular/ papular	face, moving down body	nil	post triangle lymphadenopathy arthropathy
Scarlet fever	macular/ papular	circumoral pallor	tonsillitis strawberry tongue	cervical lymphadenopathy
Chicken pox	crops of vesicles/ pustules	face and trunk mainly	mouth lesions	secondary impetigo often
Meningococcal septicaemia	petechiae ecchymoses	anywhere		collapse meningism later

PALPATION

Tenderness
bones/joints—osteomyelitis/septic arthritis
loin   —pyelonephritis
RIF   —appendicitis (fever not marked)
parotids   —mumps
liver   —hepatitis

Splenomegaly
infectious mononucleosis
malaria

Hepatomegaly
hepatitis

PERCUSSION

Chest
pneumonia
empyema

Abdomen
confirm hepatosplenomegaly

30

AUSCULTATION

Chest
pneumonia
Abdomen
peritonitis (silent)

PAEDIATRIC NEUROLOGICAL EXAMINATION

The nervous system can be examined by observing the child moving and playing in a relaxed environment. More systematic checks of reflexes and cranial nerves, for example, can be performed when you have had a chance to build the child's confidence in you.

INSPECTION/OBSERVATION

1 **Level of consciousness:**
   alert
   drowsy
   irritable
   episodic alterations—petit mal
                    —partial seizures

2 **Motor system:**
   posture
   gait
   muscle size—large in Duchenne muscular dystrophy
              —wasted in polio and cerebral palsy
   limb size   —undergrown in hemiplegia (affected side)

PALPATION

1 **Sensory:** it is best not to approach a child with a pin to test modalities of sensation in routine examination. Light touch can be assessed by gently touching the child with cotton wool or a finger, when the child's view of that area of skin is obscured.

2 **Motor:**
   muscle power
   muscle skills—neck control
              —sitting
              —walking
              —hopping

muscle tone

reflexes—absent in leg in spinal tumours
        —absent in polio affected limb
        —exaggerated in cerebral palsy
          (persistence of primitive reflexes: moro, grasp, tonic
          neck response)

PERCUSSION

The 'cracked pot' sign may be obtained in hydrocephalus

AUSCULTATION

It is worth listening to the skull to hear bruits which may emanate from arterio-venous malformations or even tumours.

Students are often asked to examine the cranial nerves. Here is a brief scheme which covers them to some degree:

I   **Smell:** sniff a hidden mint and recognize it
II   **Visual acuity:** test depending on age—see below
II   **Visual fields:** confrontation test
II,III,IV,VI
    Eye movements: following your finger and pupil light response
VIII **Hearing:** test according to age—see below
VIII **Balance:** standing on one foot/walking along a line
V   **Feeling:** tell child to close his eyes. Ask him to say when he can feel you lightly touching his face
VII Screw up eyes/puff out cheeks
X   View palate when child says 'aah'
XII Tongue movements
XI   Shrug shoulders

VISION TESTING

1 Newborn babies will fix their eyes on faces.
2 Babies of about 6 weeks smile responsively.
3 Infants from about 7 months will attempt to pick tiny coloured pellets.
4 Infants and children below 3 years can be tested using white balls of varying sizes on black sticks against a black background.

5 Children over 3 years can be tested by showing them various sized letters at a distance which they match with letters on a card in front of them.
6 Older children can read off the letters on the Schnellen chart.
7 Ophthalmoscopy—cataracts?
                —papilloedema?

SQUINTS

These can be seen by observing the reflection of a distant light source on the cornea. In the normal child, the reflection should appear symmetrically in both eyes in respect to the position of

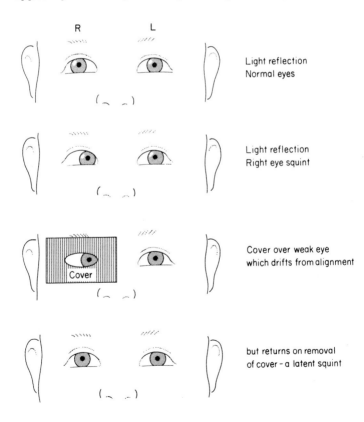

Light reflection
Normal eyes

Light reflection
Right eye squint

Cover over weak eye
which drifts from alignment

but returns on removal
of cover – a latent squint

34

the pupil. If one eye is weaker than the other, when it is covered it will drift out of alignment and return when the cover is removed.

HEARING TESTING

Babies will still to sounds or become restless when the background noise ceases.

Infants will turn their eyes or even heads to sounds when made approximately 45° behind and lateral to them. To test this, the child must be temporarily distracted by someone in front of them and then a faint noise with a high pitched rattle or a softly whispered sound is made from the appropriate position.

From two years onwards the child can be asked to hand his mother particular objects. The examiner should keep a reasonable distance, shielding his mouth to avoid lip reading.

In the older child the examiner can whisper numbers for the child to repeat.

SPEECH

Note should be taken during examination of whether there is any vocalization:

cooing
babbling
word repetition
accurate use of isolated words
linking words
sentences

and noting any pronunciation problems or stuttering.

PRECAUTION

With all these tests of development great care must be taken to avoid causing anxiety in the child or parents. Any delay in a child attaining a milestone or learning a new skill may be interpreted by the parent as evidence that the child is retarded or spastic. An isolated abnormal sign in this area proves nothing except that the test should be repeated at a later date.

THE CARDIOVASCULAR SYSTEM

As with the other systems, observation of the child playing or feeding may provide valuable diagnostic information, e.g. sweating and tachypnoea during feeding in an infant with heart failure, or squatting during exercise in a child with Fallot's tetralogy.

INSPECTION

1 **Tachypnoea and respiratory distress**
2 **Colour: central cyanosis**
   transposition of great vessels (baby)
   Fallot's tetralogy (usually older)
   respiratory causes
3 **Pallor and peripheral cyanosis**
   hypovolaemia
   poor cardiac output
   stress (e.g. pain)
   cold (NB: neonates turn red when hypothermic)
4 **Sweating**
5 **Shape and symmetry of thorax**
6 **Thoracic visible pulsation**
7 **Jugular venous pulsation**
8 **Clubbing**
9 **Peripheral oedema**—seen in infant as facial oedema and
                        excessive weight gain

PALPATION

1 **Pulse rate and volume**—low volume in hypoplastic left heart
                            syndrome, collapsing pulse in patent
                            ductus arteriosus
2 **Femoral pulses**—absent or delayed compared to radial pulse
                     in coarctation of the aorta
3 **Position of apex beat**—beware of dextrocardia (especially in
                            exams)

4 **Heaves and palpable heart sounds**
5 **Thrills or palpable murmurs**
6 **Hepatomegaly**
   evidence of heart failure
   pulsatile in tricuspid incompetence
7 **Splenomegaly**
   infective endocarditis

PERCUSSION

The smaller the child the less percussion will help in the
cardiovascular system examination. It may help to confirm
cardiomegaly or hepatomegaly.

AUSCULTATION

It is important to listen over the four main areas:

1 **Mitral**
2 **Pulmonary**
3 **Aortic**
4 **Tricuspid**

and follow any murmur heard along its maximum intensity
radiation. It is sensible to check regularly the common radiation
areas such as the neck and the left axilla. In children, some
murmurs may be heard best in the back (e.g. coarctation of aorta).

Heart sounds

Splitting of second sound is very easily heard in children
especially over the pulmonary area where P2 is delayed in
respect of A2 in inspiration. Fixed splitting is heard in atrial
septal defect (ASD). The third sound, best heard in the mitral
area, is normal in children.

Murmurs

The following features of murmurs in children can be helpful in
diagnosis and separating the pathological from the common
innocent murmur.

Timing: ejection systolic/pansystolic/continuous/diastolic
Changed by posture/respiration
Maximum at pulmonary area/left sternal edge IIIrd space etc.

Radiation to neck/axilla etc.
Loudness: often graded out of 5

Nearly all heart disease in childhood is related to congenital abnormality of the cardiovascular system. However, in the past and in some developing countries today, rheumatic heart disease contributes to the prevalence.

When considering the possible diagnosis any syndrome or other congenital abnormality should be borne in mind. For example there are recognized associations between the following syndrome and heart problems:

1 **Down's syndrome**
   ventricular septal defect (VSD) (most common)
   endocardial cushion defect
2 **Turner syndrome**
   coarctation of aorta
3 **Rubella syndrome**
   patent ductus arteriosus (PDA)
4 **William's syndrome**
   aortic stenosis (AS)—supravalvular

Table of paediatric heart problems and murmurs

	Timing	Radiation	Other signs
Innocent	systolic	nil	no thrill/alters with posture BP normal
VSD	pansystolic	all over	thrill/parasternal heave if VSD large
ASD	systolic	pulmonary	fixed splitting of second sound (murmur from pulmonary flow not from blood passing through ASD)
AS	ejection systolic	aortic neck	sudden collapse during exercise
Coarctation of aorta	often none	back	radial-femoral delay or absence of femoral pulses/hypertension

THE RESPIRATORY SYSTEM

Respiratory disease is a very common cause of illness in childhood.

INSPECTION

1 **General appearance:**
   ill looking/febrile
   reduction in activity by breathlessness
   thriving?
   patches of excema

2 **Breathing:**
   tachypnoea
   inverted timing in pneumonia
   use of accessory muscles
   grunting in expiration in preterm babies
   asymmetrical chest movements in pneumonia or
   pneumothorax

3 **Cyanosis**

4 **Clubbing**
   early clubbing may be difficult to see in small children but very
   likely in chronic bronchiectasis, usually cystic fibrosis. The
   diagram below shows how the diamond shape between two
   thumb nails tends to disappear:

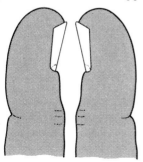

Normal

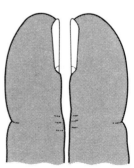

Clubbing

PALPATION

It is useful to palpate the position of the trachea in children but it may upset them, so perform this last and explain what you are doing. In pneumothorax in preterm babies a sudden apparent hepatosplenomegaly may take place as a result of these organs being pushed down by the expanding intrathoracic air volume. This may occur in severe asthma. Tactile vocal fremitis is not very helpful in very small children.

PERCUSSION

Hyper-resonance:
pneumothorax
asthma
Dullness:
over consolidated lung
over liver area which may be higher than normal if area of collapse above
Stony dullness:
pleural effusion

AUSCULTATION

Breath sounds:
decreased over effusion
decreased over pneumothorax
increased over consolidation. However in small children, expansion of the affected side during inspiration may be reduced so that breath sounds are not heard.
Vocal fremitis:
whispered 99 in older children and talking or crying in younger. Same changes as breath sounds.
Added sounds:
wheeze
crackles
   As explained under breath sounds the signs may be misleading in small children who hardly move the affected side of the chest in pneumonia so added sounds may be heard on the less affected side.

Table of signs and common chest problems in childhood

Problem	Chest movement	Percussion	Auscultation	Other
Pneumonia	reduced that side	dull	bronchial breathing medium crackles	febrile ill
Asthma	reduced but hyper-inflated	hyper-resonant	wheezes coarse crackles	atopic
Pneumothorax	unilaterally reduced	hyper-resonant	distant sounds	acute onset distress
Pleural effusion	slightly reduced unless large	stony dull	absent sounds	aegophony at upper edge

THE ABDOMEN

The positioning of the child in abdominal examination is
important. Although it is easier to elicit physical signs with the
child lying on a couch or bed, many children feel threatened by
this. It is possible to examine toddlers lying on their parent's lap
provided their heads and legs are supported to relax their
abdominal muscles.

INSPECTION

1 **General appearance:**
   thriving
   jaundice
   ill
2 **Abdominal shape:**
   Generalized distension—the 5 'F's:
   —fat (obesity)
   —fluid (ascites)
   —faeces (constipation/Hirschsprung's)
   —flatus (intestinal obstruction)
   —foetus (not to be forgotten past puberty)
   Localized distension:
   upper—pyloric stenosis
           —hepato/splenomegaly
   lower—obstructed bladder
3 **Visible peristalsis:**
   upper left to right—pyloric stenosis
   upper to lower—small intestinal obstruction
4 **Inguinal region:**
   herniae?
   lymphadenopathy?
5 **Genitalia:**
   undescended testes
   ectopic testes
   hydrocoele

phimosis

vulvovaginitis

6 **Anus:**

fissure

ectopic

With the last two areas mentioned it is vital to use tact and discretion and always have a chaperone, preferably the parent, present. In practice one considers the possibility of child sexual abuse if the history is suspicious. During clerking of patients students would be advised against perineal examination unless a member of staff had directly requested you to do this. This is not a problem with small babies but would be in older children, especially adolescents.

PALPATION

Always try to ascertain if there is likely to be any tenderness before you start to examine the abdomen. Most children over 2 years will be able to point to areas which are tender. Young children will be more cooperative if you do a mock examination of one of their toys first or if you palpate either using their hand first or putting their hand on top of yours.

The questions you are attempting to answer are:

1 **Is there guarding or tenderness?**

Where?—appendix

—hepatitis

—renal tenderness

2 **Are there abnormal masses present?**

What?—Wilm's

—neuroblastoma

—faecal loading

—intussusception

3 **Are the viscera enlarged?**

Which?—hepatomegaly

—splenomegaly

—hydronephrosis

Remember to palpate from the right iliac fossa towards the spleen and the left iliac fossa towards the liver or you may not feel the edge if the organ is grossly enlarged because you will already be on top of it.

The same recommendations apply to palpation as well as the inspection of the anus and genitalia. Although in practice rectal examination is an essential when indicated by a history of abdominal pain, etc., it is unethical to submit a child to this examination for your own practice.

PERCUSSION

To confirm the size of the organ you have palpated, and to demonstrate shifting dullness and fluid thrill of ascites. Ascites is usually caused by nephrotic syndrome in childhood.

AUSCULTATION

The bowel sounds are absent in peritonitis or a paralytic ileus following surgery or severe sepsis in infancy. They may be exaggerated in intestinal obstruction and in acute diarrhoea in gastroenteritis.

BONES AND JOINTS

ROUTINE INSPECTION

When you are watching the child with reference to the neurological state and general appearance, it is important to consider whether the child has:

A limp, possibly due to congenital dislocation of the hip. It is routine to screen for this after birth but some cases cannot be detected at this stage, therefore it is worth including this in your examination of the pre-walking infant. The instability of the flexed, adducted hip and the relocation with a 'clunk' during abduction is suggestive of a congenital dislocation—Ortolani's and Barlow's manoeuvre.

1 **Pain in the joint:**
   slipped femoral epiphysis
   Perthe's disease
   arthritis

2 **Fracture:**
   accidental
   pathological (bone tumour)
   non-accidental (child abuse)

A malformation of a limb
talipes equino vulgus/varus
congenital phocomelia
osteogenesis imperfecta
rickets

PALPATION

Before palpating a potentially tender joint or bone ask the child to point to the most tender area so you can approach this carefully. In children with joint pain get them to perform the passive movements before you test the joint movements. Your questions during examination should be:

Is there tenderness/redness/swelling?
Is there limitation of movement?
Are other bones or joints involved?
Is there associated muscle wasting? (chronic condition)
Are there signs in other systems to help distinguish between:
osteomyelitis
fractures
Henoch-Schonlein purpura
sickle cell painful crisis
osteogenic sarcoma or
Ewing's tumour
juvenile chronic arthritis?

PRESENTATION OF FINDINGS

The results of your interview with and the physical examination of your child patient should be carefully recorded on paper. Brief notes taken during the interview can be written up in full afterwards. This is good practice for your note keeping when you have qualified, practice for your final examination and is valuable for revision. If you take the opportunity of reading around the subjects which arise in the differential diagnosis and management of the children you clerk, your written record of the child's case will act as an *aide-mémoire* during revision.

When you have completed your notes it is helpful to list the major problems. This problem list will help with planning the appropriate management and will help you to keep your follow up notes in a logical order when you are attached to the paediatric wards. In an exam it will allow you to provide a rapid summary to the examiner if this is requested.

Here is an example of this approach:

PROBLEMS:

1 Vomiting
2 Weight loss
3 Maternal anxiety

DETAIL:

1 **Vomiting**
from age 4 weeks for 3 weeks
projectile
undigested milk
curds in vomit
occurring as long as 3 hours post feed
visible peristalsis
palpable pyloric tumour
2 **Weight loss**
dropped from 50th to 10th centile in 2 weeks

skin turgor reduced
sunken fontanelle
3 **Maternal anxiety**
cannot stop baby vomiting or crying
afraid that baby is going to die

PLAN:

1 Ramstedt's pyloromyotomy.
2 Intravenous infusion to correct dehydration after confirmation from checking urea and electrolytes.
3 Explain congenital pyloric stenosis to the mother and reassure her about the success of the operation and how her recognition of her baby's illness has helped the situation.

   The problem orientated approach may not be standard in your medical school but it is helpful to experiment with it.
   In presenting your findings in your finals always allow yourself enough time to organize your thoughts between completing the clerking and meeting the examiner. Try to prepare a few line summaries of the main features as an opening statement.

INVESTIGATION AND TREATMENT

A valuable but painful discipline is to commit yourself to a conclusion or diagnosis at the end of your notes. This should lead you to a more rational plan for investigation and therapy.

INVESTIGATION

Because children are so afraid of painful procedures and at an early age cannot understand their value, investigations are kept to an absolute minimum. X-rays are avoided as much as possible. This means that during your contemplation of the most useful management these precautions should be borne in mind. When suggesting a particular investigation to an examiner, be sure you have good evidence to justify it. It is impressive to hear the justification as the investigation is suggested, e.g. 'I would request a haemoglobin level and electrophoresis because this child is of Afro-Caribbean ethnic origin and has had a previous attack of severe pneumonia, septicaemia and abdominal pain.'

TREATMENT

Similarly, it is also necessary to justify the administering of any form of treatment. Many treatments have undesirable side effects, especially in childhood. If you suggest a potentially risky treatment to your examiners, you will be safe provided you explain the reason with evidence from your history or physical signs. It is also worth mentioning the side effect, e.g. 'Although corticosteroids can present a growth retardation problem in childhood, because of Jamie's repeated urgent hospital admissions and severity on arrival, together with the difficulty of administering bronchodilators to a 2 year old, I would prescribe them for a trial period.'